UNSPINNING YOUR WORLD

UNSPINNING YOUR WORLD

A Guidebook for Parents Raising a Child with Autism and other Disabilities

VIVIANA DE FELIPE

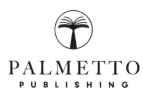

PALMETTO
PUBLISHING
Charleston, SC
www.PalmettoPublishing.com

Paperback ISBN: 979-8-8229-3459-7

INTRODUCTION

It began as a menial job in a daycare facility after relocating to Miami. The country of Peru was going through a turbulent time and my parents outlined a career path for me without giving me an opportunity to say something about it. Despite their pleadings and objections, I paused college education and made my way to the United States. My sister left a few years earlier with her new husband and settled in the city of Kendall just South of Miami. They had an extra bedroom and invited me to live with them to find my own career path.

I took any job that I could get. Working 12-hour days for almost a year in the sweltering Florida heat at a dry cleaner was the most sweat gland stimulating job I wouldn't wish on an enemy. Thankfully, my sister found a daycare center that needed a teacher. The job paid about the same but the air-conditioned classrooms sealed the deal.

I really didn't think much about this thing until I started my new teaching job at the daycare and one of my children had autism. I had some experience with autism in college. During a semester studying Psychology, our class had to do a short rotation in a Psychiatric Hospital. There were many people with all kinds of mental illnesses including a few children who were diagnosed with autism.

A child at the daycare was struggling at first but by the end of the first day he seemed to be positively responding to me. Within a couple of weeks, he was even thriving. It wasn't long before other teachers pulled me from my class to help them with a particular child with autism in their class.

So many times, I've heard teachers tell me, He has autism. Like it explained everything. It was like the child was given a long sentence in prison and they'll never make parole. My approach is simple. Children with autism are different. You simply have to learn to speak their language. It's like traveling to a country where you don't know the language. Frustrating at first, but with gestures, grunting, and some finger pointing, you eventually find a way to communicate.

It's been fifteen years since I started at the daycare. I now live in South Carolina, have two children of my own, and a Master's Degree in Psychology. I've been in the field over ten years working with special needs and children with disabilities. I've worked with hundreds and hundreds of children from two years old to eighteen years old and adults on the autism spectrum. My gift or thing or magic is really not a secret at all. It's more like someone who has an ear for languages. Maybe I have an ear for the autistic language. However, it's a language anyone can learn with the right guidance, experience, and of course practice.

One of the most interesting things I've learned on my journey is that a child with a diagnosis such as autism has to learn "our language" in a different way. They learn differently. It is usually the parents who get frustrated when they attempt to take a traditional approach to learning. It is not for us to get mad at the child who doesn't speak "our language". If we are visiting another country, would we get impatient or angry at someone in their country because they don't know how to speak our language?

The title of this book is meant to remind the parents of a child with a diagnosis or learning disability that they learn in a different way. Let me be your guide and teacher to help you navigate one the most difficult and satisfying journeys a parent can take. A journey through life with a child who has a disability.

TABLE OF CONTENTS

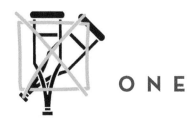 ONE

A DIAGNOSIS IS
NOT A CRUTCH

"Until you have kids with special needs you have no idea of the depth of your strength, tenacity and resourcefulness

-Anonymous

*Having a diagnosis doesn't mean your child cannot
learn to be successful and independent.*

Receiving a diagnosis for your child can be scary, overwhelming, and shocking. A thousand and one feelings and thoughts shoot through your mind and no one can prepare you for it. You'll find you need to regroup and rethink options.

Throw traditional understanding out the window and know your child learns, sees, and perceives the world around them differently. It's like learning a new language or culture of another country, only it's your child. All you really need to understand is *their* "language."

Having a diagnosis is never an excuse to stop learning or to accept certain behaviors. It's most certainly never an excuse to do nothing. Your child deserves to be successful and given the opportunity to learn and achieve their fullest potential. It's a wonderful journey and your child will surprise you. A diagnosis is not a label. It is only a part of who they are. It does not define them. It's up to you to open up the world to them so they can become their true self. I'm here to show you how.

Let's begin with some things you need to do. You must understand the diagnosis from different approaches while trying not to get discouraged from possible outcomes. I encourage you to seek out those who have a lot of experience working with children and see how they approach certain behaviors and concerns. They almost always have a different and interesting point of view. Also, talk to other families that are going through a similar experience. Seek out a local group to join (or one online) where you can connect with other families going through the same experience.

Look for as many resources as possible. Your child is unique and his treatment, therapy, and approach should be too. Understand that a person is very complex. The human body, brain, and behavior encompass so many factors that it is impossible to define it through one single approach. There's not a magic formula or a pill.

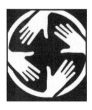 Form your own support group, you will need it. Support groups include: **Family members** (close and extended), **friends** (family friends, your friends, BFF), **professionals & experts** (people with experience in their field including Doctors, Therapists, Financial Advisors, and Lawyers), **Health and Wellness experts** (fitness instructors, coaches, counselors,

exercise groups, classes, and retreats). **Recreational Groups** (hobbies, clubs, and other classes). **Spiritual Advisors** (place of worship, spiritual leaders), **Daily helpers** (people helping with daily chores, such as cleaning, kids transportation, cooking, laundry), and don't forget about other families going through similar experiences.

Start your research and find Doctors that have experience with your child's diagnosis. Don't be afraid to get second and third opinions. Don't be afraid to look for alternative and innovative treatments and therapies. I highly recommend you seek out what different approaches others are doing. Choose the path you want to follow. Look at all resources local, in other states, even in other countries. Pay close attention to the statistics in your child's diagnosis and symptoms. Start making phone calls to those places and collect all the information available.

Ask yourself these questions:

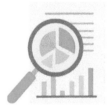

- Is there a concentration of your child's diagnosis and symptoms in different states or countries?
- What different treatments might be available?
- What are other families saying about those treatments?

Some suggestions for google search:

Resources for (diagnosis)...
Treatments for (diagnosis)…
Alternative treatments for (diagnosis)…
Experts in these treatments for (diagnosis)…
Books on these treatments for (diagnosis)…
Innovating therapies for (diagnosis)…
Best country to treat (diagnosis)…
Prevalence of (diagnosis) around the world.
Statistics of (diagnosis) in other countries.
Statistics of (diagnosis) in other states.
Books on (diagnosis).
Experts on (diagnosis).

Here's an example: If we look at the most prevalent cases of autism on a global scale, the United Kingdom is ranked 1st in the world. The United States is 4th behind Sweden and Japan.

As research continues and other approaches increase with diagnosis, several other alternatives and innovative therapies have emerged such as sensory integration, animal therapy, diet modifications, exercise routines, transcranial magnetic stimulation and much more.

A person cannot be defined with one approach. Having a diagnosis can affect the person as a whole. Therefore, having different approaches considering how it can affect the person as a whole may involve exploring and utilizing different approaches, therapies, and treatments.

Look at this guidebook as a type of roadmap to help you organize your thoughts to find the right path for you. I do not know your child's diagnosis. Therefore, I cannot give you an exact treatment plan. You should consider this guidebook as a way to better help you speak your child's language and give you insights on how to ask questions getting you closer to a treatment plan your child needs.

You will need to become an expert on your child's diagnosis. You need to continuously research options outside your state or even your country to see what others are doing. Explore *all* possible options. Be proactive.

There is usually a long waiting list for treatment services. Years can go by before a child can receive services. Sometimes a child will even age out of the system. Unless you have extensive resources, a child will not receive any therapy during this critical time in their lives. This guidebook is designed to jump start this process.

Research possible ideas you can do at home with your child now. There are things you can do to promote growth and skill acquisition while you are waiting to receive therapy. Start working on a plan of action that will probably be in constant motion and change as you find more information and your child grows and flourishes. Nobody knows your child better than you. Nobody has your child's best interest in mind more than you. Trust your instincts and don't be afraid to fight and ask for what you believe your child deserves. Acceptance is not an option.

HONESTLY ANSWER THIS QUESTION:

 How would you describe your life at this moment? How do you want it to be better?

CONTACT LOG SHEET

AGENCY/ORGANIZATION	DISCIPLINE/Profession	CONTACT INFORMATION (Name, phone, email address)

CONTACT LOG SHEET TRACK

DATE	AGENCY	INDIVIDUAL NAME	NOTES	FOLLOW UP

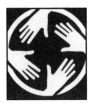

YOUR SUPPORT NETWORK

Write down names of people that belong to each of your support groups as explained in this chapter.

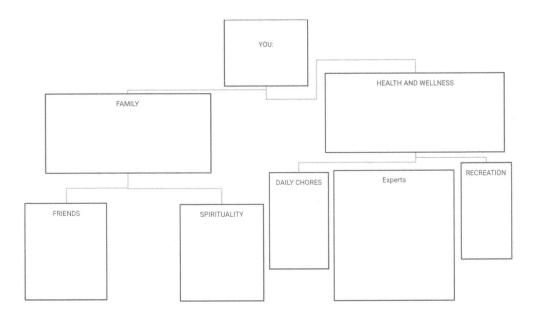

TO DO LIST BEFORE MEETING WITH PROFESSIONALS

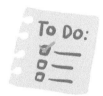

Below highlights some of the activities to complete ahead of time along with materials to bring to your meeting with a professional.

- Prepare questions for the team and list them in order of priority.
- Prepare a goal plan along with any questions.
- Prepare a preliminary list of services you think may be appropriate.
- Ask about referrals, options, and any of the processes.
- Review the results of any assessments, reports, and screenings.
- Underline questions, concerns, and progress (or lack of) observed and recorded.
- Invite additional participants (any individuals you think may be helpful) to be there with you. These are people that may have helpful input, questions, and can provide emotional support.
- List what you want to accomplish by the end of the meeting.

What to bring to a Meeting:

- All the material and notes listed above.
- Notebook and pen.
- Any recent assessments, reports, or screenings.
- Any new approach, service, or research that you may think will be beneficial with any questions you may have.

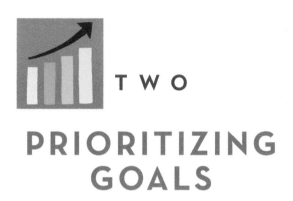

TWO

PRIORITIZING GOALS

"It shouldn't matter how slowly a child learns. What matters is that we encourage them to never stop trying."

-Robert John Meehan

Formulate goals for your child, your family, and yourself.

Think about your family's schedule. Consider a daily routine which will keep the family unit balanced as a whole. It's important to create a blend which functions around all family members. Pay close attention everyone receives the attention they require to maintain a harmonious environment. The goal is to find a routine that works with everyone in the family.

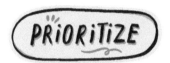

Once you have these answers, you can formulate and prioritize your goals. Begin with one or two goals at first and build on that. Think about what will be most important or urgent. Meet with your support group and team of professionals to get their input on what will work to reach your goals. Evaluate how much time you are able to dedicate to work towards those goals and how much effort and commitment you need to invest. Then decide on a plan to best fit with your family's needs.

Once you have educated yourself and have learned more about your child's diagnosis, you will be better armed with resources and a support team to start looking and trying different treatments and/or therapies. Remember that these are decisions made as a team in collaboration with the professional team. Always ask questions, challenge your professional team so that you understand the reasons behind their suggestions and you can make an informed decision.

The following pages contain several questions which will be helpful to have in mind when thinking about goals. HONESTLY ANSWER THE QUESTIONS

Fill out the sheet as completely as possible.

List your child's likes and interests:

List your child's dislikes:

List your child's strengths:

List the skills your child has:

List the challenges impacting your child's life:

What would you like to see change with your child and the family unit?

What would you like to see your child do more of or less of?

What are your short term goals? What do you need to change now?

What goals do you want to achieve in the next 3 to 6 months?

What are the long-term goals for your child?

For example: Living arrangements, education, work, vocational training, and social networking.

List the things that have worked successfully with your child:

List of things you have tried that have been unsuccessful.

What is your availability? Make a sample schedule of your daily activities.

What is your commitment?

Write days per week, hours per day, and times of the day which work best for you to dedicate specific time to work on your goals

Another factor to keep in mind is that working on things will be more difficult and overwhelming for you rather than your child. You have to be prepared to cope with the consequences and behavior that may stem from challenging your child. This is not meant to discourage. It is to prepare you to make an informed decision and commit to the plan. You must be prepared for possible consequences. Sometimes when you introduce changes, things look tougher in the beginning. However, if you stick to the plan, things will start going better.

BREATHE

There is never a stupid question and you have the right to ask anything and everything you think you need to know

Each time you meet with a professional team or provider, make notes about what you would like help with along with any concerns you have. Include what you want to learn and to accomplish. Talk to as many people and professionals as you can. The more information and opinions you have the better-informed decision you can make. Remember, when you meet with experts and professionals you are also interviewing *them*. Your goal is to find the ones that you think will fit best with your family's needs and values. There is nothing wrong with making an informed decision or changing your mind along the way.

THREE

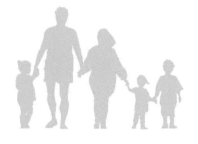

QUALITY FAMILY TIME

"As special needs parents we don't have the power to make life "fair," but we do have the power to make life joyful."

ANONYMOUS

Having a child with a diagnosis can consume all your time and thoughts if you let it.

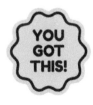

Don't forget to spend quality time with yourself, with every member of your family, and make time for your personal relationships. Some parents may feel guilty spending time away from their children. They believe it takes away focus from the child.

Parents wear many hats: Husband, Wife, Mother, Father, and friend. It's OK to have quality time with each and don't forget yourself as well. If you don't allow time for yourself and the other important people in your life, you will get burned out. Some may even start developing feelings of resentment. Relationships need attention and time to grow to keep flourishing. It's not fair to you and the other people around you to provide the attention they need as well.

If you start feeling resentment or get burned out, you will not be able to help your child and build the important relationships in your life. Especially with the one you have with yourself. If you want to help your child effectively and have a healthy family relationship, you need to be in a place to provide the attention and quality they crave and need. It is important to focus on quality time with the entire family. It might seem difficult at first but you'll find your way and the family dynamic will thrive.

A child with a diagnosis may need extra attention, but you have to make time for your other family members as well. Create opportunities for the whole family to participate. After all, you want that family unit to remain intact and be happy. A diagnosis is not a wedge to separate the family unit and you never want anyone in your family to perceive anyone as a burden or an obstacle.

One great strategy is to include the entire family in therapy and treatment discussions. Let them contribute and be involved. This will give everyone an understanding of the treatment and can be involved in it. They'll thrive and be excited knowing what role they can play or would like to play.

Another great strategy is to find activities your whole family can participate in and enjoy. It can be simple things to do at home or add to the daily routine. If you're wondering what you can do, don't worry. I've made a list of some examples which can help.

Here's a list of suggestions which can increase the probability of a positive response.

On set Activity	Examples	Skills / activities	To do	Prepare in advance
Playing games/ interacting with family	❑ Reading books ❑ Board game ❑ Matching game ❑ blocks/Legos ❑ Puzzles ❑ Popping bubbles ❑ Tag ❑ Catch ball	• Social interactions: Completing an activity together • Following instructions • Social/leisure activities- taking turns, sharing • social communication	• Explain the activity (clear and simple instructions) • Explain the rules before starting activity • We need to play together until • Use a timer to give him a visual of the duration of activity. • Explain rewards & consequences • Once we finish, we can... First-then • Give choices (do you want matching game or puzzle) • Tell your child how she did and Give rewards	• Be sure you have all needed supplies/materials needed to complete activity. • i.e. timer, reinforcement chart, books, puzzles, games etc.

Area	Activities	Skills	To do	Prepare in advance
Activities to do while sitting at the table with family E.g meal times at home, restaurants, etc	❑ Eating ❑ Reading books or magazines ❑ Playing games ❑ Puzzles ❑ School work	• Eating together- soc interaction • Completing an activity together- social interaction • Following instructions • Working on responsibility (school work)	• Explain the activity (clear and simple instructions) • Use a timer to give him a visual of the duration of activity. • Explain the rules • We need to stay at the table • Explain rewards & consequences (Once we finish you can....) First-Then statements • Give choices • Tell your child how he did and Give rewards	• Be sure you have all needed supplies/ materials needed to complete activity. • i.e. timer, books, puzzles, worksheets, pencils etc.

First/then statements - ('then' = the activity they like)

A **Reward** is a verbal statement and/or gesture which encourages, promotes, and acknowledges your child's achievements and/or participation. For example: "It was so nice doing (activity) with you. I really enjoy our time together. Thank you for spending time with me. Thank you for helping me (activity). I am proud of you for trying (activity). It's great you completed (the activity).

The **reward** can also be the activity they originally like/wanted to do - OR - the completion of the activity requested. It should be delivered along with the verbal statements as described above.

FOUR

BUBBLE WRAP

"All kids need is a little help,
a little hope, and someone who
believes in them"

-Magic Johnson

If only we could wrap our kids in bubble wrap to keep them safe.

Reality is something different. In the long run, we know it's certainly not practical or beneficial. It is our responsibility as parents to prepare our children as much as possible for what life may throw at them. Adaptability and flexibility are very important skills to have. One thing's for sure, life changes all the time and we cannot control it. Adaptability is key to being as independent as possible.

It seems to be easier to "give-in" to your child's wants and make them "happy" in the moment. Ask yourself: Will this prepare your child for the impending changes that you won't be able to control?

Starting early with small changes will build a better foundation for the changing world coming their way. The longer you wait, the more rigid and inflexible habits they will form making it difficult for them to change or adapt.

Flexibility and adaptability is a skill you will *always* be working on. Consult with your team of professionals. Keep track and observe how your child is responding and progressing with their adaptability skills.

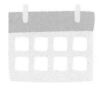

Challenging them shouldn't put down their confidence. Work to built them up to make them stronger. Everybody has different capabilities, strengths and weaknesses. Use their strengths to push them to the next level. Build on the strengths so their skills will help improve their weaknesses. We all have the potential to achieve our goals. We may need to use alternative methods. Search for creative and unique ways to get there.

Structure can be very helpful for you and your child. It will allow you to manage the appointments, house chores, meetings, work, dates, etc. Balance time between all family members, your friends, and your important relationships.

An organized schedule can be very beneficial and provide flexibility. It doesn't need to be rigid. Allow room for changes and the unexpected. Learning to cope with change is good training to strengthen and build on flexibility skills. This can also serve as an example for your child. They will learn important skills to build and use a schedule as they make their way through life. An organized schedule can be one of the most important skills your child and family will use.

Simple things can be life changing and will allow you to have quality time. Seamlessly going different places, waiting in line, being with different caregivers, or doing different activities throughout the day can be life altering.

Here's an easy way to change up the daily routine. Use baby steps to teach them flexibility. Instead of one parent always doing the bedtime routine, change it up and rotate family members, read different books, eat at a different table, or walk a different route.

As parents, we want to protect our kids from anything and everything. The reality is we want them to be prepared for life. We won't be around forever and need to make sure they are as prepared as possible. We must teach them how to adapt and respond to an ever-changing world. They must learn to cope with as much change as possible. Teaching moments may not be the easiest ones and sometimes they don't feel good while we're applying them. As long as you have your child's best interest in mind and build on their strengths and confidence, you are doing what you think is best to prepare them for life...

Pat yourself on the back - you are being a great parent!

Understand, you cannot control everything in your child's life. There are simply too many factors out of your control. As difficult as it will be, it is better to prepare them for the many possibilities that life will throw their way.

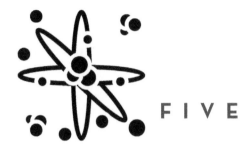

FIVE

ACTIONS & REACTIONS

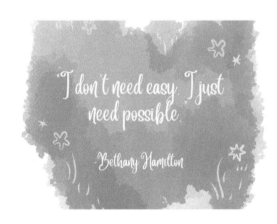

"I don't need easy. I just need possible."

-Bethany Hamilton

Depending on which perspective or approach you have with your child, there may be a new "meaning" which may help you understand things from different points of view.

We've all been "punished" by our parents growing up. Most of us have "punished" our kids at some point. The idea behind punishment is to stop or decrease the probability that our children will behave in the same manner.

Sometimes this doesn't quite work the way we intended. It might work for a while, then the behavior we were trying to stop happens again and we come up with a more intense punishment. Punishment is a reaction to our child's behavior. A child's behavior after the "punishment" will be the result of your reaction. This turns into a cycle of actions and reactions between parents and children's behaviors.

There are different approaches that can be used to stop this cycle of reactions. They can be used in combination or separately depending on your goals, keeping in mind your child's strengths, personality, behavior, and weaknesses.

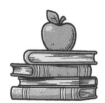

One method is to teach a more appropriate behavior to obtain the same original result instead of using the undesirable behavior. It is very important that you observe and decipher what your child is trying to tell you when they use these types of behaviors. Once you are able to identify what your child wants to accomplish, you can teach them a more appropriate way to behave that will give them the result they are looking for.

When your child learns a different (more appropriate) behavior that replaces the undesirable behavior by giving them the same outcome, there will be no need to use the undesirable behavior. This will create a longer lasting skill and will help reduce those undesirable behaviors while giving them the tools and skills they need to be successful. In other words, we focus on increasing and teaching more appropriate behaviors instead of the undesirable behavior.

Let's look at a case with Kevin as an example. He was 13 years old and couldn't speak. One of the behaviors his Mother was concerned about was hitting himself on the chest or the head seemingly for no reason. She didn't recognize why Kevin was getting upset and this was his response.

Everyone tried to keep Kevin as calm as possible without upsetting him so he wouldn't hit himself. This became stressful for the family, especially for his Mother.

After documenting several observation sessions in his behavior journal, we discovered Kevin hit himself when he was asked to do something he didn't want to do or when he wanted to stop an activity.

Our solution was to teach Kevin to sign for "stop" and "no." Next, we taught him to use the appropriate sign when he wanted to stop an activity or didn't want to do something he was asked to do. We implemented several control opportunities (manipulated choices and environment) to give him choices we knew he didn't like in a specific way which allowed us to teach him to say "no" or "stop." In those specific situations when he would usually engage in inappropriate behaviors, we stopped him and guided him to sign his response.

Once he mastered signing, Kevin was able to indicate "stop" or "no" instead of beating on himself.

NOTE: Everyone has come across a child *acting up*, being silly, or doing things they're not supposed to be doing. These behaviors usually happen when you are having a conversation with other adults (Read... when your attention is focused on something else besides the child). To get your attention, the child will climb furniture, cry, spill juice, or any other inappropriate behavior to gain your attention - positively or negatively. We all have heard the expression "acting out," or "putting a show for others," or "he is usually not this way."

Children crave attention from their caregivers. Children do not discriminate "positive" attention from "negative" attention. For them, any type of attention is attention no matter if you are hugging them, or you are screaming at them to "stop it." As long as they steer the caregiver or parent's attention towards them, it doesn't matter if the attention comes in the form of screaming, chasing, or playing a game.

Something similar happens in certain instances when we react to a child's behavior by giving them attention through yelling. We may have just given them the attention they were looking for and therefore *increase* the possibility of those behaviors to happen.

Sometimes when we think we are using a form of punishment with the purpose of stopping or decreasing a behavior, we may be *encouraging* or even *increasing* the probability that similar behaviors will continue.

According to some behavior and learning principles, behaviors can be learned and/or modified according to our experiences. If a child is looking for attention and acts or behaves in a way to obtain it and the response/reaction they get from those actions is the attention, they learn those types of behaviors will result in the outcome they were looking for - the attention. Therefore, next time they want attention, guess what they will do? The reaction towards your child's behavior will teach them how to behave next time in a similar situation.

It is important to think before we react to our children's behavior.

The lesson we may be teaching might be the opposite of what we intended. This task may seem impossible at times but it is better to stop and take a breath before we decide what we are going to do. Patience and observation are going to be key traits in this journey. Having a journal (included in this guidebook) is designed for you to keep track of behaviors and reactions and help identify potential patterns. Understanding actions and reactions within this perspective can help you promote more positive changes allowing you to make better informed decisions about your actions and reactions. Consider sharing the information you document in this guidebook from your observations with your support team. You want everyone to see your observations and learn what is working. Allow them to learn which behaviors might work for them as well.

Let's talk about little Evan. He was 3 years old when we first met. One of his parents' main concerns was that he constantly hit and head bumped people at the house, including his mother. When Evan displayed this behavior, his mother and other family member's reaction was to reprimand and say things like "stop that, that hurt," or "that is mean."

This was the attention he was looking for and he learned every time he wanted attention all he had to do was to start hitting, bumping, slapping, and head-butting others for what they thought was "no apparent reason."

My advice was: Every time Evan started behaving like that, instead of reprimanding him, ask family members to focus their attention on something else besides him. An example would be to start talking to someone else, head for the kitchen and wash dishes, or go do the laundry. At first, he started hitting more and at times harder. I told the parents to take a deep breath and keep the attention somewhere else. It was also fine to move to a different area - as long as everyone is safe. *

If a child starts behaving in a manner that is not safe, like climbing a chair, you MUST step in and remove the child from the chair. Avoid eye contact and don't say anything, remain silent. Then, place the child in a safe place away from the chair (sit on the chair to stop them from climbing again) or take the child to another area where there is nothing they can potentially use in an unsafe way.

* SAFETY IS PRIORITY! You will have to determine how this can be applied to your child depending on their own characteristics.

Since we decipher that what Evan wanted was attention, while doing these different strategies, we also determined what we needed to teach Evan when he needed or wanted attention. We decided to teach him the phrase "Mama look." When Evan was doing something else rather than the undesirable behavior of hitting, Mom would get to his level, say "Mama look" and give him positive attention for a few seconds. Repeating the phrase encouraged Evan to repeat the phrase and Mom gave Evan positive attention for another couple of seconds. During the day Mom made it a point to repeat that phrase and give Evan attention several times a day.

Little by little Evan learned this new behavior by saying the phrase "Mama look" instead of hitting.

If Evan started to cry, I advised his mom to go down to his level, comfort him with a little touch. If Evan started to console, Mom explained "if you want Mom, you need to say "Mama look" with no hitting. I also told her to encourage Evan to repeat it and then give positive attention.

If mom went to console Evan and his reaction was to slap, turn away, or scream, then Mom should step away for a few seconds and try again.

His Mother mentioned there were times when Evan would have to wait for her attention. In this case, she will signal Evan by pointing a finger and saying "wait." She will then count to ten and afterward provide a glimpse of positive attention around every 30 seconds. A positive glimpse can be an eye wink, a wave, a smile, a touch on the shoulder, or a pat on the head.

The gap between those glimpses of attention increased as Evan learned that he will receive the attention he needed and learn to tolerate not having attention for longer periods of time.

This is an illustration of how seeing, understanding and dissecting behavior of others and ourselves, and seeing behavior from different points of views can change the way we react. This allows us to implement "outside the box" strategies to explore different outcomes.

Another concept to keep in mind is natural consequence. This is a concept which may require an understanding of abstract concepts as the child matures. One of the ultimate goals is for your child to understand their actions have consequences and how those consequences translate to social rules. This is an important skill and concept because it's a major component of how society works. We want our kids to understand how their actions may affect their outcomes and to break away from relying on the prompts from others.

An example would be if a child throws a toy and breaks it because he was mad or too excited. Instead of buying a new toy or attempting to fix it right away, allow the child to calm down and explain to them that toys may break if they throw them. Teach your child a more appropriate and acceptable way to express their emotions which will help create correlations between their actions and the consequences.

If you present a task like no TV before a reading or homework assignment, OR no TV after 8:00 pm, give them reminders of the time especially if the assignment is not being done. If the assignment is not completed before 8:00 pm because they chose not to do it or do something else, then you will have to follow through and enforce the rule of no TV after 8pm.

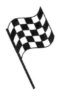

This is the beginning of teaching your child the essential skills they will need later in life. Children need to learn and understand how their actions and reactions affect others and the consequences of their actions. Another example would be following rules and understanding consequences of their actions in the workplace. This can translate into project due dates, punctuality, behavior with colleagues, and workplace procedures.

Learning the appropriate way to behave socially and social manners will be most beneficial and important. We can start teaching these during childhood so children will have the time they need to learn this at their own pace and they can acquire the skills necessary to be as independent as possible.

They can start learning their actions have consequences and there are social rules we need to be aware of. This may seem far-fetched in the beginning but it is an important skill that can be taught at different age levels and can gradually be acquired over time.

Be prepared! When teaching this skill, your child will push back and give you attitude. Remember how reactions to behaviors work with different perspectives between you and your child. Be careful not to set your child up for failure. You want to be sure they have the tools needed to succeed while doing the task. Make sure you are teaching skills they need and provide consistent guidance. Patience will be a virtue; the teaching period can be long and repetitive.

Encourage your children to ask for help if needed. Help them by guiding and supporting them but do NOT do the task for them.

The tone of your voice will also affect the type of response you get. Some children need a monotone or a flatter way of speaking while others a tone that implies fun and excitement.

Presenting a request as a choice can also help. It gives the illusion parents are giving up control. In reality, giving them options maintains control because you control the options to increase the probability, they will choose what you prefer. You can give them the option to pick the place where they would like to do their homework by suggesting - either the dining room table or in their bedroom, and what homework to start with - either science or math.

Instead of saying "Do your homework" and getting resistance, it gives the illusion that it was your child's idea and on their terms.

Don't forget to encourage, appreciate, and show gratitude to your child. Acknowledging their accomplishments and showing appreciation may seem small but it has a BIG impact. Encouragement promotes growth & learning and they'll appreciate you more with your positive words.

For some reason, we all tend to pay more attention to negative behaviors than the positive ones. Changing this will not only improve the relationship with your child, it will help improve relationships with family members and friends. Always look for a more positive way to see and approach situations.

You cannot control the behaviors of others. You can only control yours and certain parts of your environment. Use them to strategize your actions and reactions. You will then be able to teach and modify the desirable behavior and increase the behavior outcome you desire.

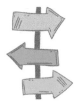

Another thing I have observed in children who are displaying an episode or a moment is their "fight or flight" response trigger. If we step in aggressively, yelling, or giving them big gestures like screaming "stop" or "you are grounded," the fight or flight response will either make your child's behavior increase or they will run away from you. If you go in calm from a protective and helpful approach saying things like…

"I'm here to help,"
"Let me help you so you won't get hurt,"
"Tell me what you need so I can help,"

…in a calm voice and no big gestures, the fight or flight response usually diminishes and your child will relax, allowing you the opportunity to teach.

Examples of behaviors Journal

Child's Actions	Parents reaction	Child's actions	Parents reaction	Child's actions	Lesson
Screams or cries when they want ice cream	Screams and yells "no" then takes away toy	Child keeps asking for ice cream. Child gets louder and more intense	Gives child ice cream (Parent wanting to stop the crying and screaming)	Child stops screaming	Parents appeased the child to stop the screaming by giving ice cream The child learned: If I Scream and cry long enough eventually I get what I want

Parents Actions	Child's reactions	Parent actions	Child reactions	Parent actions	Lesson*
iPad or phone off at bedtime	Defiant refusing saying"no" ignoring parents' instructions	Yelling, making threats, taking away other things, not giving back, grounding, etc. Trying to snatch phone or iPad away	Keep playing with phone or iPad, resists parents snatching and/or running away	Parents give in and allow extra time on the device or allows them to take the ipad to bed	Parent: Fighting stopped once comprise was granted Child: If I resist long enough I get what I want

* This doesn't mean that negotiations and compromises are wrong. It is actually a good cognitive skill to have. Parents are the ones who should give the options and stay in control of the negotiations and compromises and not the child. Negotiations are better to start during the first phase of these interactions so the child learns at the beginning there is a better or more appropriate way to communicate.

Keeping track

Child's actions	Parents reaction	Child's actions	Parents reaction	Child's actions	Lesson

Keeping track

Child's actions	Parents reaction	Child's actions	Parents reaction	Child's actions	Lesson

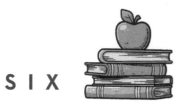

SIX

SCHOOL STUFF

"Teaching kids to count is fine, but teaching them what counts is best"

-Bob Talbert

Get as much information as possible.

Do as much research as possible. Your child has rights and parents have rights as well. You are the only one that can advocate for your child and demand what you think is best for them and the best way is to get informed.

There are a few things that can be helpful when deciding what school route to take. Common choices are public school, charter school, private school or home school.

Research all schools. Talk to other parents and read every review. Meet with the administration and teachers. Be sure to ask about the curriculum and more importantly, their knowledge of your child's disability. See what resources they offer for parents and children with disabilities. See if they understand what the best setting is for your child during the day; what will they do to make your child succeed in school; what role you want school to have in your child's life; what is the school's long-term goal; what is the purpose of your child's education; and, how will a school setting help them accomplish their goals.

Whatever route you choose, make sure you are well informed. Have a clear idea of your rights and the rights of your child. Ask for a copy of their policies or procedure manual. See if they will be a good match for your child. Public schools have certain rules and regulations they have to follow under state education law and regulations. Be sure you are familiar with those as well. Public schools are sometimes less flexible in some of their procedures because there are more administrative steps involved and more regulations that need to be followed to consider certain types of services and or requests. It is helpful if you ask about disciplinary policies and how they will be applied to your child.

Private schools can be more flexible if they are open to accommodating children with special needs. However, this is not always the case. Some private schools may not be equipped, trained or have the resources to provide certain accommodations due to their policies and regulations. This is why you need to get familiar with them and ask questions about their policies regarding accommodations, goals, resources, disciplinary actions, crisis management, and any other important topics relating to your child.

Charter schools may also be another good option as long as they are prepared to accommodate special needs children. They can also be more flexible about accepting other agencies who can go to the school and provide the resources they are not able to. Depending on your child's skill level and needs, Charter schools may provide a mainstream educational setting with additional accommodations that are not available or too difficult for public schools.

Educate yourself! The best way to find out what will be best for your child is by researching and meeting with potential schools in your area. Get as much information as you can find, consult with special needs education lawyers and search for resources they have available. You will find some of these options won't be a good fit. You will also find one or combination of some that are.

Homeschooling is another great option. Note that each state has their own rules, regulations, and policies they need to follow in order to be in compliance.

To find the right homeschool options in your state. search homeschool laws and regulations in your state and their associations and coops. They can help you with resources and with the documentation you need to stay in compliance.

A secret weapon is a homeschool tutor. They can be very helpful providing your child with the specific instruction they need. Keep in mind it might be difficult for some children to see you as the teacher instead as "Mom". This can create some confrontation and frustration. A tutor can keep those roles separate and decrease confrontation which will allow you to maintain a healthy relationship with your child. You can also find online homeschool options, and hybrid homeschool models that would help reduce the frustration of teaching your child making school a more positive experience. Another perk of homeschooling is, depending on your state regulations, you can choose the curriculum to teach along with how and what to teach as long as you keep records of the required documentation and complying with the minimum core class requirements.

IMPORTANT!

To help guide you, which education route will work best for your child, write down a comparison chart with the different options they offer and what they don't. Have a list of departments and the people in charge you may need to speak with about different accommodations and services. Write down short term and long-term goals you would like your child to achieve in school along with the support they will need to reach those goals. Through careful examination, you will discover which type of school will be most beneficial for your child.

See next page for example of the school comparison table, contact log, and communication log.

Here is a list of some of the contacts you might find helpful in your educational quest:

Teachers, teacher's assistants, behavior support specialists, special education coordinators, principals, speech therapists, occupational/physical therapists and their directors, directors of the psychology departments, counselors, assistant technology directors, and online groups - just to name a few.)

IMPORTANT! Always keep a record of who you make contact with and the reason for the contact. Be sure to write down what you discussed along with their responses. Below is a **School Contact Log** which will help keep you organized.

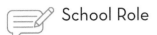

School Role

What role you want school to have in your child's life; what is the school's long-term goal; what is the purpose of your child's education; and, how will a school setting help them accomplish their goals.

School comparison sheet

School name	Experience with diagnosis	Resources and accommodations	Disciplinary policies	Values, culture, view of disabilities	purpose, goals

✎ SCHOOL CONTACT LOG

School Name:

NAME	DEPARTMENT	CONTACT INFORMATION (phone, email)
	Teacher	
	Principal	
	Special Ed coordinator	
	Psychology/counseling	
	Behavior specialist department	
	Speech therapy	
	Assistive technology	
	Occupational therapy	

School Communication LOG

Date	Person contacted	Reason	Response and date

SEVEN

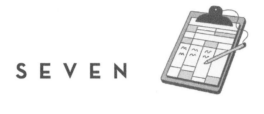

EDUCATIONAL PLANS

INDIVIDUALIZED, THE 504, AND THE TRANSITION PLAN

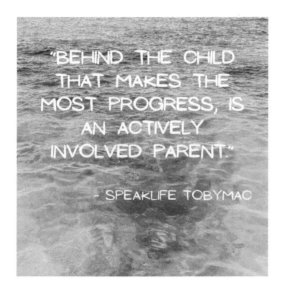

"BEHIND THE CHILD THAT MAKES THE MOST PROGRESS, IS AN ACTIVELY INVOLVED PARENT."

- SPEAKLIFE TOBYMAC

You have the right to request an IEP, 504, or BIP Plan.
What is an IEP, 504, or BIP Plan?

Get familiar with the options and services available along with the processes you will need to follow to request those services. As a parent, you *are* the advocate for your child. The end goal would be to teach your child to advocate for themselves to the best of their capacity. However, in the beginning, you will always be the advocate no matter their age or abilities.

 ## THE PLANS EXPLAINED

The IEP (Individualized Education Plan)

This is a legal document that contains evaluation results, eligibility criteria, present skill levels, education goals, accommodation, and other services like speech, occupational or physical therapy, service hours, and how those are provided directly or indirectly, type of curriculum and standardized testing criteria.

The thirteen eligibility categories are: *Autism Deafness, Deaf-blindness, Hearing impairment, Mental retardation, Multiple disabilities, Orthopedic impairment, other health impairment, Serious emotional disturbance, Specific learning disability, Speech or language impairment, Traumatic brain injury, Visual impairment, including blindness.* *

Students meet the criteria if they have at least one of the thirteen categories and their disability has a negative educational impact on their educational performance. Educational performance includes academic, social, emotional, and their behavioral outcomes. A child can be in a regular classroom setting and still have an IEP. Having an IEP does NOT mean the student needs to be in a self-contained special education classroom. It only means the student has a specific plan of education with goals and accommodations specific to their learning style.

To be eligible for special education, a child must have a disability and must need special education services and related services. If a child has a disability but does not need special education services, the child is not eligible for special education under I.D.E.A. but may be eligible for protections under Section 504 of the Rehabilitation Act. (www.wrightslaw.com)

The IEP will state the type of curriculum the child would be learning, either a modified, adaptive or regular curriculum, a list of the accommodations the child will need to be successful in the school setting, as well as the type of standardized testing the student will be participating in. Some students in special education are exempt from standardized testing. You can also request to have specific accommodation for testing based on the accommodation.

Some accommodations may include: Visual aids, small group testing, use of fidgets, use of augmentative alternative speech devices, additional prompts & instructions, breaking assignments into smaller sections, frequent attention, additional breaks, sensory breaks, use of calming area and or sensory area.

Make sure you know what works for your child and how your child learns. You are the one that will request those accommodations. Make sure they are written in the plan so the school is held accountable. No matter how simple, small, or common you or the school thinks their accommodations are, **be sure they are written in the plan.**

The 504 Plan

Section 504 is a civil rights law that prohibits discrimination against individuals with disabilities. Section 504 ensures that the child with a disability has equal access to an education. The child may receive accommodations and modifications. Unlike the Individuals with Disabilities Education Act (IDEA), Section 504 does not require a public school to provide an Individualized Educational Program (IEP) that meets a child's unique needs and provides the child with educational benefit. Under Section 504, fewer procedural safeguards are available to the child with a disability and the child's parents than under IDEA. (www.wrightslaw.com)

This document states specific accommodations your child will need in the school setting. This is used when a child doesn't qualify for an IEP or special education services. The child attends regular education classroom settings with a set of specific accommodations which will allow them to be successful at school.

Examples of these accommodations are: Additional time for assignments and testing, small group testing, use of fidgets, additional breaks, and a personalized visual schedule.

Behavior Intervention Plan (BIP)

This is a behavior plan put in place to address a specific targeted behavior. This is something parents can request (I usually recommend it) if the child gets frequent notes sent home or phone calls from the school about their behavior.

This is a process that can take several weeks. I suggest you start as soon as you get the first notes or phone call about their behavior. An IEP will be conducted to make the request. Once the request is signed by the parent, the school will coordinate with the school psychologist or behavior specialist to conduct an FBA (functional behavior assessment) to determine the function of the behavior, potential triggers, targeted behaviors, and possible strategies. A team will meet to discuss results and decide if a BIP needs to be put in place if they agree a BIP is needed. Next, the team will have a meeting to put the BIP together and revise strategies suggested by the psychologist/behavior specialist. This will include behavior data collection, specific strategies, and behavior targeted goals.

NOTE: Be sure to request access to the behavior data so you can keep track of your child's progress.

The use of a "*shadow*", *educational aid* is sometimes an option. If a child needs additional support besides what the classroom setting offers, a shadow or educational aide can be allotted. Parents can call an IEP meeting to request this accommodation. The important part is the team must agree there is enough supportive documentation to suggest this is necessary for the child to have appropriate educational services in the least restrictive environment.

NOTE: Some accommodations and requests may be difficult to obtain. Some schools may push back, make excuses thinking it is not necessary or it will take too long to coordinate the accommodations. In the meantime, your child may remain in an environment that is not good for their success. This is where it's important to know the law, regulations, and have a special education lawyer that can help you navigate through this process. It puts you in a position to put pressure on the schools if necessary. You can also look for parent advocates and IEP consultants that will help you navigate the process as well. They can go to the IEP meetings with you to advocate for your child.

Transition IEP

This is conducted the year your child turns 13 years old. This plan discusses the potential high school paths the student will follow to reach their goals and prepare them for life after their graduation. Don't forget to plan for the future! What will happen after high school? What would be the best path for them to follow?

An important suggestion is to talk to the teacher before the IEP is in place. Your child will probably be invited to participate. If you want to be the first person to talk to your child about their participation, make sure this is discussed with the teacher.

 Document in writing information for the teachers so everyone knows what to expect and how to handle these circumstances. You are allowed to opt-out your child from participation if you feel it's in their best interest. If you believe your child has the ability to participate, have a conversation with them first explaining what to expect from the meeting and see how they feel about it.

Most children appreciate their inclusion and are glad to participate in the meeting. After all, it is their education and their future so it is important to let them have a say in what their goals and dreams are for their future. Remember, during the IEP, the diagnosis will be brought up. If your child doesn't know about it, it will be best to have that conversation first and explain it to them so they are better prepared for the meeting. This is also a good time to get together with your team of professionals to see what will be the best way to approach this conversation and what type of resources there are which can help explain this to your child and make it easier to understand.

Different paths to explore depending on future goals

The most common are a High School Diploma, a job certificate, or an attendance certificate.

High School Diploma: This is a standard diploma from High School. If your child started in a differentiating setting or path but was able to end his education in a regular edition setting, they can receive a high school diploma.

Job Certificate: Students in this setting attend a self-contained classroom with modified curriculum that concentrates on job skill acquisition. The goal is to prepare them to be employable citizens. Some schools will have a vocational liaison which can assess students and see if they are eligible for job placement. Students receive an employment certification stating they have completed employment courses and can work regular employment hours. The vocational liaison can help find employment which meets your child's needs and may be able to provide training for the job.

Attendance Certificate: Students attend school in a self-contained classroom and receive a modified curriculum mainly focusing on daily living skills. At graduation they will receive an attendance certificate stating they attended a high school program.

If you have specific questions related to your child about a specific situation with the school, reach out to me at viviana@sproutforkids.com

Future Plans

Questions to think about and to discuss with your child. Where possible, let your child answer most of these questions.

 What are your dreams for the future? (For example, 1, 2, and 5 years from now)

What would you like to do after high school? (College, trade school, work, day program, workshop, where would you like to live, have your own_____etc

Is there something about the future that worries you or concerns you?

Who are you? How would you describe yourself? What do you like about yourself? What are your strengths, gifts, talents? What are your dislikes?

What do you like to do? Activities, themes, hobbies, subjects etc.

What do you think you need to achieve or accomplish to reach your dreams? What skills do you think you will need to reach your goals?

Who can help you with your plans for the future? Who can help guide you to obtain the skills you need and reach your goals?

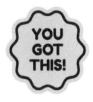

Use these answers to formulate a plan which will be the most helpful and beneficial to give your child the skills they need to achieve their future dreams. Also, use these answers to formulate their IEP goals including their long term goals. The IEP should reflect the skills gained to reach them as well. Address the needs and make the necessary adjustments which will help them reach their goals.

There are due dates and an order of events which need to be followed when conducting a valid IEP and 504 plan including when and who is informed and participated. Be sure you are familiar with those rules. Parent advocates in your area are a good resource to find out those rules and make sure your IEP is in compliance. It is helpful to talk with your team of professionals and therapists to have an understanding of strategies and techniques that work with your child; and especially, the ones that haven't. You can use these recommendations as a base to create needed accommodations in school that are specific to your child.

Make sure all accommodations are written and documented clearly in the IEP and it is shared with all of your child's teachers. They should have a clear understanding of the accommodations they need to implement.

In my opinion, going to an IEP with people in your support system is very helpful. Parent advocates are helpful with the processes and rules for compliance and will help you navigate the different services and how to make the requests.

Having people from your professional team - such as therapists and caregivers - can help bring another layer of support and information about your child to implement strategies that have been successful. Your support team can also make sure the IEP goals are tailored to your child's specific needs and their long-term goals. You as a parent can invite anybody that you feel will be important to have in those meetings.

It is important for parents to know that if at any point you feel your child is not receiving the appropriate services, there is documentation of lack of progress, multiple attempts of trying to resolve the issue without getting results, you can always request a meeting with district staff or consult with your special education lawyer to seek a solution.

Your child can spend a large amount of time in the school setting. Twelve years, five days a week, eight hours a day is over seventeen thousand hours for them to learn academic, social, emotional, and behavior skills. It has to be as productive and beneficial for them as possible.

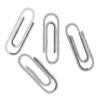

EIGHT

UGH, PUBERTY

Note to self:

When things feel overwhelming, remember:

- One thought at a time
- One task at a time
- One day at a time

It can be scary and begin sooner than expected.

A diagnosis can affect the onset of puberty in children. It can start sooner or be delayed. In some cases, pre-puberty can start as early as 9-10 years old. It can also be accompanied by behavioral symptoms such as irritability, moodiness, emotional, restlessness, and increased impulsiveness. Some parents have reported more talking back, making hurtful or mean comments, not listening, aggressiveness to self and others, lethargy, sadness, unmotivated, or loss of interest in things that were interesting before. Children can display some or all of these behaviors sporadically and without apparent pattern or reason. **This is why it is so important to keep a behavior or observation journal. It can help to get a better** **understanding of your child's development.**

You may observe your child struggling or behaving differently towards you or others for an unusual period of time. During these times, they may be a little more moody or emotional. Think of it this way, we all have times when we are out of sorts. It usually lasts a day or two and we return to feeling more like our regular selves. Children also go through these cycles or it could be an indication that they may not be feeling well. When this happens, observe and document the change. If it continues for several days consult with your doctor to rule out any potential illness or physiological reasons. If those are ruled out it may be the possibility that pre-pubescent or puberty symptoms seeping in.

Your child will grow and enter a new phase in their life. As scary as this may sound it can also be exciting. Don't panic! You can prepare yourself for the upcoming changes. Talk to your pediatrician and get as much information on what to expect along with the options there are to pursue depending on what your child will need.

You're not going to like this BUT it is also a good time to discuss possible birth control methods with your doctor. They are turning into adults and unfortunately it may be time to explore what options are available. This will allow you to make educated decisions on how to proceed when you think it's time.

Don't forget to talk with your professional support group how this may affect what changes may occur and what goals and treatment plans need to be addressed with these new behaviors. It's so very important for parents to be informed and have a plan of action ready for this inevitability. Don't forget the children need to be explained and taught the changes in their bodies and what those changes mean. Be sure to address this with your team of professionals and, importantly, with family members so everyone is on the same page.

Make sure you agree with the information before you share it and follow how the information is delivered.

Some important topics to consider during this stage in life are hygiene, grooming, healthy eating habits, relationships, girlfriends, boyfriends, masturbation (if this is something your child starts displaying) and with girls, their menstrual cycle. There are several books and social stories on these topics. Personalized social stories are a great way to talk about these topics. They can be tailored to your child's level of understanding and make it easier for them to relate to the information. Talk to your team of professionals about creating a social story with the topics you need help with. Don't forget about the internet. You can search endlessly for a thousand social stories. Zero in one the ones that will help you best. There are also several sites that offer plenty of examples you might be able to customize. Many are free but some may require some form of payment.

I know this is not a preferred topic which parents want to discuss, especially at earlier ages. However, just like the sun will rise, it is something that is going to happen no matter what. Everyone is affected by this stage of life differently but we all make it through. Everyone goes through puberty no matter the diagnosis or skill level. The way it affects them is different for everybody but it can correlates with their characteristics and personality.

This is something that cannot be ignored or pretend will not happen. It 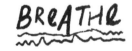 is better to be educated and have a plan on how to handle it. Be sure to include your professional and support team so everyone knows how to address this new phase. It's OK to lean on them for the support you need. That's what they are there for.

I can't express enough how ignoring this will catch up to you! It might be difficult to address this situation in a way you feel comfortable but waiting will give you less time to prepare and get information and once the genie is out of the bottle, it will be more difficult to control.

You need to understand and be prepared for the inevitable changes and unexpected circumstances that will catch you by surprise and understand no matter how prepared in advance you are, you won't be entirely prepared. The best you can do is educate yourself so you can minimize those surprises and be prepared as much as possible. Get ahead of it. Having more time to get ready will allow you to handle the situation when it rears its ugly head.

NINE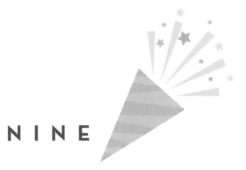

DON'T FORGET
TO CELEBRATE

"Success is not final,
failure is not fatal: it is
the courage to continue
that counts."

-Winston Churchill

The more you celebrate your life, the more life you have to celebrate.

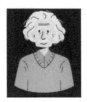

Einstein once wrote on a chalkboard the multiple tables for the number 9 from 1 to 12. When he wrote 98 as the answer to 9 x 11, the classroom ribbed him about the incorrect answer. He humorously asked them why they didn't praise him for the eleven he got right?

I urge you to see the cup half full instead of half empty. Human nature has a bad habit of focusing on the negative: Things we don't like or are not what we want. Life with your special child will have its peaks and valleys. So what - that's life no matter your circumstances. You are on this wonderful journey together and the journey will be so rewarding. Your child will change and grow in different ways. So will you. Your child will learn differently. So will you. That's a great thing.

Think about your day and all the things you complain about. How many negative thoughts found you? Now turn that around and think about all your accomplishments no matter how small:

POSITIVE VIBES

You woke up! You walked to the bathroom. There was hot water in the shower. You put on nice clean clothes. There was food in the refrigerator and you had quality time over breakfast with your family. You had a nice conversation on the way to school. You went to your job because someone sees value in having you as part of their company. Simple things of course. Why celebrate something we do every day, day in and day out. When negativity creeps in replace it with something to be grateful for and as quick as possible. You'll soon find you're in a happier state of being.

Remember the old saying: "If Momma's happy, everybody's happy."

Which type of reflection and focus makes you feel happier and less stressed? How do you think this will affect your attitude towards others? What type of attitude do you think will allow you to have a healthier relationship with family and friends?

Focus on the positive progress and accomplishments - no matter how small. If you feel you're not making progress, your child will sense it and believe they are disappointing you. Your attitude towards the situation will reflect your interactions with your child and the family.

Celebrate any accomplishment! There is no small accomplishment, just an accomplishment. Celebrate the progress of moving forward. Celebrate their new word or word approximation, using a gesture to ask for something, controlling emotions in a tough situation, not having a potty accident in a day, putting their shoes on by themselves. There are so many things in a day to celebrate. You just need to make the effort to look for them. This will create a less stressed, fun environment in which everyone wants to participate in and be a part of.

It might sound difficult but it's not. It's a simple mind shift. A habit that is worth changing and learning. All you do is shift the thought from negative to positive. When you feel a negative thought coming on, recognize it and make a quick shift to something positive. Before long you won't even know you're in the habit until you feel happier.

YOU'VE TOTALLY GOT THIS!

Life throws enough bad energy at us on a daily basis. Tune it out. Take the time and make the effort to adopt this important skill. Your support group can also be a helpful guide. You will have rough days and struggle to get into that positive mindset. Reach out and get in touch with your support network, your friends, family, health wellness, spiritual groups. They can be a great resource if you need a pick me up type of intervention.

Remember to celebrate together.

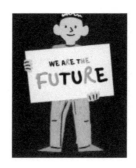

T E N

PLANNING FOR
THEIR FUTURE

Every child deserves a
champion: an adult: who will
never give up on them, who
understands the power of
connection and insists they
become the best they can
possibly be."

- Rita Pierson, Educator

It's always in front of us and can never be seen.

The future is a tricky place. It can seem far away or a little too close. It may seem difficult to plan because of so many unknown things. Be cautious! Having a plan with urgency may reduce the possibility of different options. Take your time.

 Planning for your child's future can be stressful, scary, and uncertain. This is why it is important to begin thinking about potential plans. Just as plans are not set in stone as your child grows and acquires different skills, your situation can and will change. Members of your support network will change also. Don't be afraid to change a member that doesn't have the best interest of the group in mind or seems to be more of a negative influence. As life goes, you might have to relocate the family to another city or state and you may find yourself replacing your group entirely. The internet can also help keep you in touch with some people that are in a similar situation, meetups, Facebook groups etc. are a good way to find resources and connect with others that are going through similar situations as yours. Just navigate the internet with caution. The point is… you have lots of options.

It's always a good time to start creating a plan of action for the future. Don't worry how plans might change. They will. Be flexible to modify the plans depending on how things develop but work on getting a plan for the future in place.

 Your goal is to help your child acquire the skills they need to be successful in whatever environment they may be. Many have gone on to successfully receive college degrees either attending regular classes or adaptive college.

Clemson University's LIFE or College of Charleston's REACH programs are geared for special students. Here are some questions you'll need to consider if you plan for the future education of your child: Will they be living on campus or commuting? Will they look for employment? If so, what type of employment? Will they be attending a day program? Will they remain living at home with family members or head into a residential program? What type of care will they need?

As your child grows and learns, paths and options may vary and can be modified. It is better to start thinking about the future so you can work with your team to teach your child the skills they will need to be successful in any of the settings and environments they will find themselves in.

This is why it is important to teach your child the skills they'll need to be as independent as possible and reach their full potential. The sooner you start, the more time you have to teach them the necessary lifelong skills. This is the main focus of early intervention and why it is so important. Begin observing right away and nurture them through the skills they're going to need to give them the best chance for success.

Receiving Therapy Services

Receiving services can be unpredictable and frustrating. This doesn't mean you cannot start working on a plan. Reach out to your support group. Someone usually has a great idea for alternative therapies. Be proactive. If one provider is not available, look for others who are. Sign up for every waiting list you can find. Worst case scenario… if you're selected, you can always say you don't need them at this time.

This goes for any therapies, residential settings, and living arrangements you may think you need and those you're not sure of. A common example is the residential setting. This is an option that takes years on a waiting list. In my experience, it's better to research options as soon as possible, even if you've just signed up. If it turns out your child won't need this type of care, you can simply decline services or take your name off the waiting list. At the least, you'll have options instead of waiting until you need it and there's nothing available.

Another thing to keep in mind, be prepared when your child turns 18 years old. At this age they become legal adults and you will not have access to medical records, school records, or a say in medical treatments and even their money management - unless you have a Power of Attorney or a legal guardianship.

   If you think your child will need help with these types of decisions, you will need to get legal counsel to proceed with the legal process to explore options and make an informed decision that is in the best needs of your child. Depending on your child's limitations and strengths, there are different options for how you can structure his affairs. Options include - but are not limited to - guardianship, conservatorship, or power of attorney.

Guardianship is the most restrictive. The person assigned as the guardian will make all decisions regarding your child. Your child will not be able to have input on any of the decisions regarding his living situation, medical treatments, who he is allowed to see, and his money management - just to name a few.

A Power of Attorney covers decisions regarding medical treatments and living arrangements among other legal matters. Parents can offer input and guidance and be involved in the decision making process, reviewing relevant documents and information, but the ultimate decision will come from the child. There are several ways to set this up depending on the needs of the child. Talk with your lawyer and get the advice and information you need to make the best decision and how to proceed.

Begin this process before your child turns eighteen! This can be a lengthy process and you don't want to be in a situation where your child turns eighteen and there is a gap in which doctors won't be able to share information - or - you won't be able to make decisions regarding schools, medical treatment, and other matters.

Keep in mind there is an instrument known as a limited power of attorney. This document involves decisions only for specific matters.

Don't forget about the Financial Arrangements

Align yourself with legal and financial experts to advise you about the best options to utilize so your child can receive the services they need. Special needs consultants, lawyers, and financial advisers are the best professionals who can help you explore these options. Some available options are: A special needs trust, estate planning, and eligibility for government benefits. There are many different options to explore depending on your situation. Don't be afraid to go down every road you can think of to get the services your child needs. Talk to other parents, join local special needs groups, talk to your doctor, physical therapist, or other provider and grill them about what they're doing.

In Summary...

Having a plan early in the process and being informed will pay off in the long run. Start thinking about the future NOW! Begin formulating a plan as far ahead as possible so you'll be prepared.

This brings us back to being proactive. Research all available options you think will be the best fit for your child. Don't discount the little things you can implement at home. Participating in family time activities are important opportunities to work with your child and teach them the social skills they're going to need (see chart above on family quality time chart).

This guidebook is designed to organize your life with your special child. I've included many blank pages to organize your thoughts and keep track of your child and their progress all in one place. I've formulated specific questions I've been asked by the thousands of families I've worked with.

The real secret weapon will be your support team. Be selective who you want to have in your inner circle. Other parents with special needs are an obvious choice. You might also consider your pediatrician, physical therapist, General Practitioner, or other therapists. Also keep in mind the world is at your fingertips. In the age of the internet, you might find the best qualified professional in France, Iceland, or Bangladesh. Join other groups on social media and start picking their brains.

When you begin to create a plan of action for your child with a diagnosis, don't forget to plug in your family. Your family is the most important part of your inner circle. Everyone is part of the family unit and must be included. Don't forget about you as well.

This book will help you organize your flow of information so you can create a successful plan encompassing the many factors involved in having a child with special needs. It will help you prioritize your goals so you can find the best solutions and how to best achieve your goals.

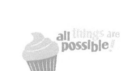

The journey is the best part. Love will carry you through the difficult times. All you have is today, enjoy every minute of it.

This book is a culmination of my experience working with thousands of children from all over the spectrum and diagnoses. In a unique twist, I find myself more and more guiding the parents of these special people. It is my hope this guidebook will help you weave through the maze of this journey with your child giving you a better perspective of what life looks like through *their* eyes.

Think of this workbook as a kind of Rosetta Stone. However... you have to actively participate in learning their language. Imagine how great your lives will be when you can speak their language and guide them to be the independent and successful individuals they can be. It's what we all want for our children.

I created this book for parents to give them a starting point on the journey ahead. The intent is to give them the tools they need to support their children to reach their full potential, increase quality of life and maintain healthy family relationships. I believe parents should be empowered to lead this journey. Parents need to surround themselves with people and professionals who can teach you tools you will need. At times, you'll feel like things are out of control. This guidebook is designed to help prepare you for the journey ahead. Get ready to make changes and take control!

If you have comments or concerns or need clarification on anything you've read or don't completely understand in any part of this workbook,

If you would like me to be part of your support group as one of the professionals to guide you and support along the way,
reach out to me at:
viviana@sproutforkids.com

I'll answer any questions to the best of my knowledge or point you in the right direction for any other information you might need.

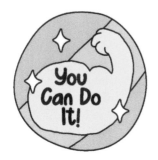

To DO or not to DO
with Diets and Meds

There seem to be endless questions about medications, diets, and other nontraditional medical approaches. What will be better, what will work, what should I do? These are questions that most parents have and the answer is not simple. I've had parents battle with guilt and failure when trying something and it doesn't give the results they're looking for. Finding answers takes time and a lot of trial & error. Don't give up! Try several approaches until you find the right ones that work for your child. As long as you are searching for the best option that's in your child's best interest, you are doing what every great parent can do.

When choosing a path, I suggest looking at the pros and cons, side effects, time and commitment. Make a list of your options, talk with specialists and your support team. Decide what will best fit your child's needs. I prefer to begin with options where in the worst-case scenario nothing will happen so there's nothing to lose. However, always weigh the risk vs. benefit and choose the ones that have or are less risk. Remember, the benefits should always outweigh the risks.

A suggestion: No matter what approach you want to try, it is important you do this with the advice from experts in their specific fields.

MEDICATIONS

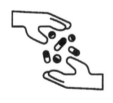

First let me give you a disclaimer: I am not a medical professional and this is not a professional opinion. I'm giving you my personal observation from working with thousands of children in the field. You must always consult with your doctor, field experts, and those in your support team when making sensitive decisions regarding this topic.

I prefer to try the more natural options first before any type of synthetic or man-made chemicals and medications. My reasoning is that a more natural approach has virtually no side effects.

Medications that come with a long list of side effects can have serious ramifications later in life. In addition, I've noticed some need to be on a regimen of different medications to deal with side effects. Another problem is when they build a tolerance. Dosages have to be increased or additional medications have to be added. This can create a cycle of long-term medication intake.

Medications are sometimes perceived as a "better" option or the first thing a doctor will recommend. They can be presented as a "better" solution because they may act quickly with less demand for work and commitment. It seems some medications may not treat the root of the problem and become a type of Band-Aid for some of the symptoms. A Band-Aid that can bring additional problems in the long run. This can lead to increased dosages or additional medications to keep covering symptoms.

I have worked with families that wanted to try medications as a temporary fix. They went in with a mindset that it is only for a short period of time with a plan to reduce or eliminate the use of the medication while they were searching for other options.

Depending on the type of diagnosis and treatment, you must do your homework to find the one that suits your child's situation. I do believe there are diagnoses that will need medications and you may find that medication is a better choice. However, be sure to ask lots of questions, consult with different people, do your own research and come to your own conclusions.

DIET & NUTRITION

We've all heard the saying, "You are what you eat." As you know, nutrition and diet have an effect on our body and will affect the way we behave. Sure, our body needs fuel to function. This fuel comes from our diet and nutrition. Depending on what type of fuel we give our body has a direct effect on how it functions which affects how we act and respond. This is the idea behind the diet and nutrition approach.

The most common foods removed from a diet to help improve behavior, mental health, and learning issues are the BIG THREE: Sugar, wheat, and dairy. There is extensive research that shows how these foods affect the function of our bodies, therefore our behavior. There's also a lot of research that correlates gut issues with mental health and learning problems.

A FEW THINGS ABOUT DIETING

Be sure you have professionals on your team specialized in your child's diagnosis like a nutritionist and a natural/homeopathic Doctor. They can outline a diet which focuses on your child's specific needs. This will require documenting patterns and lifestyle along with laboratory blood tests.

When you implement the diet and nutrition approach, I suggest you include your entire family as part of the same diet. When you cut out refined sugar, remove it from the house. There might be some grumbling from other family members but this will allow you to decrease the probability of breaking the diet. This will reduce confrontation with a child that cannot have the items they want. If other family members are eating them or if they're still visible in the cabinet or refrigerator, the child may feel they're being punished which may trigger a response. That aside, it's better for the whole family if everyone's eating healthier.

There are several very good dietary options available. Be aware most are "one size fits all" type of diet. An individualized plan is much better than a generic one. The needs of your child and family are unique to their own characteristics. In summary, I believe nutrition correlates with mental health.

Once you make a choice, commit to it! Be consistent. Positive results will soon follow. Make sure your whole team is on the same page. Your support team is also a great resource to bounce ideas, listen to their professional opinion, and help you figure out cons and pros as well.

There is really no wrong or right answer when it comes to this topic. This is a journey. Depending how your journey evolves, be aware the needs may change as well. Always ask what the expectation is, what you are supposed to observe and be looking for, any signs that you need to be aware of, or concern, timeline on what to expect, take your time to research, read reviews, and make informed decisions.

You are the Captain of this journey.
Don't forget to lead and enjoy the ride.

Milton Keynes UK
Ingram Content Group UK Ltd.
UKHW022324200324
439690UK00004B/49